W0007522

The Best Bath Recipes 500 Recipes vol.3

Logan Brown

Copyright © 2021 Logan Brown

All rights reserved.

CONTENTS

Stop! You're consuming poison every day!
Why should you buy "The Best Bath Recipes" ?
It is a collection of 500 recipes on how to make bath products, and save money.
The products will be totally homemade and 100% pure.
100% natural, fresh ingredients - You will look, feel, and act healthier than ever!

The Recipes

Oils

373. Anti-cellulite Massage Oil

Base oil:
Almond oil--2 tablespoons Carrot--5 drops
Jojoba--5 drops

Blend well.

374. Essential oil blend:

Fennel--8 drops
Grapefruit--14 drops
Lemon--8 drops
Blend well. Then add to base oil blend. Blend well.

375. Blossom Groves Massage Oil

8 tsp. grapeseed oil
6 drops orange blossom oil
2 drops lemongrass oil
2 drops neroli oil
This is a citrus-scented massage oil. Blend ingredients well. Pour into a small bottle and seal well. Warm up oil before doing any massage.

376. Crescent Moon Massage Oil

10 tsp. wheat germ oil 6 drops chamomile oil 4 drops neroli oil
2 drops rose oil

1 drop basil oil
This is a green-scented massage oil. Blend ingredients well. Pour into a small bottle and seal well. Warm up oil before doing any massage.

377. Cleansing Body Polisher with Olive Oil

1 cup fine sea salt
1/2 cup olive oil
1/2 cup melted M&P from Wal-Mart
1/2 tsp.. peppermint essential oil
This one I just mixed all together. It made a thick paste (when it
set up) that I put in a wide mouth jar to dip out with your fingers. I
think I would use this more as a foot scrub or a hand/body scrub, but not on my face.

378. Cleansing Body Polisher with Jojoba Oil

1 cup fine sea salt
1/2 cup jojoba
1/2 cup liquid soap
1/2 tsp.. orange essential oil
I poured about 1 1/2 cups of boiling water over a bunch of grated
homemade soap. I stirred it and smushed it until it cooled off

enough to mush it with my hands. Then I poured it through one of those cone shaped colanders (used for canning) with the petistal (sp?) that comes to a point at the end. I pushed it through the strainer and then strained

it again, this time removing most of the remaining soap particles. Then I measured 1/2 cup of the liquid to use in the Body Polisher recipe. This one came out liquidy and would work best in a plastic bottle with a flip top lid so you could pour it.

379. Diuretic Massage Oil:

Fennel--10 drops Grapefruit--12 drops

Juniper--8 drops

380. DreamTouch Massage Oil

4 drops Clary Sage
3 drops Ylang Ylang
5 drops Neroli
Place in 1/4 cup fractionated coconut or your favorite carrier, then rub slowly and softly.

381. Dysmenorrhea Massage Oil

Chamomile Roman--10 drops Chamomile German--10 drops Clary Sage--15 drops Fennel--10 drops Marjoram--5 drops Mugwort--10 drops Lavender--25 drops

Dilute in 4 ozs of Evening of Primrose. Massage the uterine region. May diffuse undiluted.

382. Echoes of the Wild Massage Oil

10 tsp. safflower oil
5 drops orange blossom oil
2 drops sandalwood oil
2 drops jasmine oil
This is a citrus-scented massage oil. Blend ingredients well. Pour into a small bottle and seal well. Warm up oil before doing any massage.

383. Erotic Massage Oil - Arabian Nights

Coriander 3 drops Frankincense 3 drops Lime 2 drops
Rose 2 drops

Add to 25ml base oil.

384. Erotic Massage Oil - Velvet Seduction

Rose 2 drops Sandalwood 5 drops Ylang Ylang 2 drops Add to 25ml base oil.

385. Exotic Patchouli Massage Oil

10 tsp. grapeseed oil 7 drops patchouli oil 4 drops jasmine oil
2 drops rose oil

This is a woodsy-scented massage oil. Blend ingredients well. Pour into a small bottle and seal well. Warm up oil before doing any massage.

386. Erotic Massage Oil - Sultry Nights and Roses

Geranium 3 drops Patchouli 2 drops Rose 3 drops

Add to 25ml base oil.

387. Exquisite Sandalwood Massage Oil

8-10 tsp. grapeseed oil 6 drops sandalwood oil
2 drops lavender oil
2 drops rosewood oil

2 drops rose oil
This is a woodsy-scented massage oil. Blend ingredients well. Pour into a small bottle and seal well. Warm up oil before doing any massage.

388. Exhaustion during Pregnancy.

Coriander--8 drops
Grapefruit--8 drops
Lavender--8 drops
Use 6 drops in a bath; 6 drops in 2 teaspoons carrier oil for a body massage; or 5 drops in a bowl of hot water for a foot bath.

389. Fall Harvest Massage Oil

12 tsp. grapeseed oil 6 drops bergamot oil 2 drops cardamom oil 2 drops jasmine oil

1 drop orange blossom oil
This is a citrus-scented massage oil. Blend
ingredients well. Pour into a small bottle and
seal well. Warm up oil before doing any
massage.

390. Falling Stars Body Mist

2 cups distilled water
3 tbs. vodka
5 drops lavender essential oil
10 drops chamomile essential oil
10 drops valerian essential oil
Mix all the ingredients together in a spray
bottle, shake well. Allow to settle for at least 12
hours. Store in a cool dry place.

391. Fat Attack Massage Oils: Are made by
combining:
30 drops essential oil blend
2 tablespoons almond oil

10 drops of carrot oil
Blend the almond and carrot oil together before
blending in the essential oils.

392. Forest Nights Massage Oil

10 tsp. grapeseed oil
5 drops rosewood oil
2 drops cedarwood oil
2 drops chamomile oil
This is a woodsy-scented massage oil. Blend
ingredients well. Pour into a small bottle and

seal well. Warm up oil before doing any massage.

393. Fruity Herb Massage Oil

Ingredients:
1/2 cup of walnut oil
1 Tablespoon of grated grapefruit
1 teaspoon dried rosemary
1 teaspoon dried basil
Instructions:
Put all of the ingredients together in a small saucepan and heat gently on the stove top. Do not let your mixture get to boiling point. Then once the mixture is combined, let it cool down completely. Once cool, pour the mix into a sealable jar and leave it to rest for about one week, then strain the mixture to be rid of all the the grapefruit pieces and then pour the mix into a bottle and its ready for use.

394. General Fat Attack Massage Oil:

Cypress--10 drops Grapefruit--8 drops Oregano--2 drops Rosemary--10 drops

395. Headache (Hormonal) Formula

Chamomile Roman--2 drop Chamomile Blue--2 drop Geranium--4 drops Myrtle--2 drops Nutmeg--1 drop

Sage--3 drops Spearmint--1 drop Dilute in 1 oz carrier oil.

396. Manly Massage Oil

Ingredients:
1/4 cup of mineral oil
1/8 cup of castor oil
1/8 cup of sweet almond oil
6 drops of sandalwood oil
4 drops of bay oil
3 drops of bergamot oil
2 drops of lime oil
Instructions:
Pour all ingredients into a bottle and shake well until all is blended. And shake the bottle well again before using.

397. Massage Oil

For trouble spots
2 Tbsp Carrier Oil
10 drops Lavender
8 drops Rosemary
4 drops Ginger
3 drops Peppermint
Store in a dark bottle. Shake bottle before using in the morning and evening.

398. MASSAGE OIL

1 qt. oil (from list)
4 to 8 drops essential oil (optional)
1 oz. herbs (from list)
Combine ingredients and bring to a boil in a glass or enamel pan. Simmer 20 minutes, then cool. Strain through a double layer of

cheesecloth. Add essential oil for scent, if desired. Store in a labeled, light-proof bottle. Oils Corn, safflower, soy, olive, peanut, apricot kernel, almond, avocado or walnut, or any combination Herbs for dry skin: Alfalfa, rose, chamomile
for oily skin: Lemongrass, witch hazel, marigold
for stimulation: Peppermint, rosemary, thyme
for relaxation: Sage, catnip, chamomile

399. Menopausal Sweats

Grapefruit--10 drops
Lime--10 drops
Sage--7 drops
Thyme--3 drops
Dilute in 2 tablespoons carrier oil. Massage all over the body and use 5 drops of the blend in a daily bath.

400. Minty Fresh Massage Oil

10 tsp. grapeseed oil
3 drops eucalyptus oil
4 drops rosemary oil
2 drops peppermint oil
This is a green-scented massage oil. Blend ingredients well. Pour into a small bottle and seal well. Warm up oil before doing any massage.

401. Night Dreams Massage Oil

10 tsp. grapeseed oil
6 drops chamomile oil

4 drops jasmine oil
2 drops rose oil
1 drop lavender oil
This is a floral-scented massage oil. Blend ingredients well. Pour into a small bottle and seal well. Warm up oil before doing any massage. **402. Oriental Delight Massage Oil**
Ingredients:
8 teaspoons of peanut oil
6 drops of orange oil
2 drops sandalwood oil
2 drops rosemary oil
1 drop jasmine oil
Instructions:
Thoroughly mix all of the ingredients together, by placing them all in a sealable bottle or jar and shaking vigorously.

403. Passage of India Massage Oil

10 tsp. grapeseed oil
7 drops sandalwood oil
2 drops orange oil
2 drops rose oil
1 drop cinnamon oil
This is a spicy-scented massage oil. Blend ingredients well. Pour into a

small bottle and seal well. Warm up oil before doing any massage.

404. Pina Colada Massage Oil

1/4 Cup Castor Oil
1/4 Cup Sweet Almond Oil
1/2 Cup Mineral Oil
1/4 teaspoon Coconut Fragrance Oil
1/4 teaspoon Pineapple Fragrance Oil
Combine all ingredients in a bottle and shake gently until well blended. Shake before each use

405. PMS Massage Oil

Carrot Seed--5 drops
Clary Sage--10 drops
Fennel 10--drops
Lavender--20 drops
Marjoram--30 drops
Mugwort--5 drops
Rosewood--20 drops
Dilute in 4 ozs of carrier and massage as needed.

406. Post-pregnancy Depression #1

Geranium--6 drops
Grapefruit--15 drops
Neroli--8 drops
Use up to 25 drops in 2 tablespoons massage oil (or dab on as a perfume); 3 drops in a room diffuser; or 6 drops in a bath.

407. Post-pregnancy Depression #2

Geranium--8 drops
Grapefruit--10 drops
Mandarin--6 drops

Use up to 25 drops in 2 tablespoons massage oil (or dab on as a perfume); 3 drops in a room diffuser; or 6 drops in a bath.

408. Pre-menstrual Blend

10 Drops Geranium
15 Drops Lavender
5 Drops German Chamomile
3 Drops Cypress
Place essential oils in 4 oz of fractionated coconut or your favorite carrier oil. Rub on abdomen as necessary. Patch Test of course.

409. Sensuous Massage Oil

Choose 3 or 4 oils from these oils: Clary Sage, Geranium, Grapefruit, Jasmine Absolute, Mandarin, Myrrh, Neroli, Orange Sweet, Patchouli, Petitgrain, Rose, Sandalwood, Vanilla, Vetiver, and Ylang-Ylang.
For your carrier oils, choose from Jojoba, Macadamia Nut, Sesame, or Sweet

Almond.
The ratio is 15 drops essential oils to 1 oz of carrier oil.
In a colored glass bottle, add your essential oils starting with base notes,

working up to top notes. Top off with carrier oil. Gently shake the bottle to mix the oils.

410. Sexual Energy Oil #1:

Cardamom--2 drop
Ginger--4 drops
Patchouli--5 drops
Sandalwood--4 drops
Dilute in 1/2 oz carrier oil. Wear to attract
sexual partners.

411. Sexual Energy Oil #2

Jasmine--3 drops
Sandalwood--3 drops
Tangerine--4 drops
Ylang Ylang--5 drops
Diffuse or dilute in 1 oz carrier oil for massage.

412. Solid Chocolate Massaging Bars

Ingredients:
1/2 cup of melted cocoa butter
1 Tablespoon of bees wax
1 Tablespoon of coconut oil
Instructions:
Melt the cocoa butter, bees wax and the
coconut oil in a double boiler and then mix the
oils well to combine them. Then remove from
the heat and let the mixture cool just a little to
release some of the heat. Before it is too
cool pour the mixture into candy molds and
allow it to continue cooling over night. These
bars are have a chocolatey aroma and are solid
when they are at room temperature but melt
easily at body temperature, when rubbed in
your hands. To use your bar rub it in your
hands and the bar will start to melt

and you can then use it to share a massage or on freshly shaved legs.

413. Soothing Sensations Massage Oil

10 tsp. safflower oil
5 drops lavender oil
2 drops violet oil
2 drops chamomile oil
2 drops frankincense oil
This is a floral-scented massage oil. Blend ingredients well. Pour into a small bottle and seal well. Warm up oil before doing any massage.

414. Spice of Life Massage Oil

10 tsp. olive oil
6 drops ginger oil
4 drops jasmine oil
2 drops orange oil
This is a spicy-scented massage oil. Blend ingredients well. Pour into a small bottle and seal well. Warm up oil before doing any massage.

415. Stretch Mark Oil

Rose--4 drops Rosemary--1 drop Camellia Oil--1/2 teaspoon

Sesame Oil--1/2 teaspoon Vitamin E Oil--1/2 teaspoon Wheat Germ Oil--1/2 teaspoon Massage on stretch mark area.

416. Summer Rain Massage Oil

6-8 tsp. grapeseed oil
6 drops lavender oil
2 drops rose oil
2 drops jasmine oil
This is a floral-scented massage oil. Blend ingredients well. Pour into a small bottle and seal well. Warm up oil before doing any massage.

417. Tea Tree Temptations Massage Oil

8 tsp. grapeseed oil
6 drops jasmine oil
2 drops tea tree oil
2 drops neroli oil
This is a spicy-scented massage oil. Blend ingredients well. Pour into a small bottle and seal well. Warm up oil before doing any massage.

418. Vanilla Massage Oil

Ingredients:
1 cup of grape seed oil
1/2 teaspoon of vanilla oil
Instructions:
Simply blend the two oils together by putting them both into a bottle and shaking the bottle vigorously. Then just shake the bottle well again, before each use.

419. Vegetable Oils

Apply any of the following vegetable, seed or nut oils to the skin a) Virgin olive oil
b) Sesame oil
c) Peanut oil

d) Avocado oil

420. Wild Fields Massage Oil

6-8 tsp. grapeseed oil
6 drops chamomile oil
2 drops rose oil
2 drops rosemary oil
This is a green-scented massage oil. Blend ingredients well. Pour into a small bottle and seal well. Warm up oil before doing any massage.

Misc.

421. AGING SKIN FIGHTER

2 tsp. plain yogurt 1/2 tsp. honey
1/2 tsp. lemon juice 3 capsules vitamin E

(equivalent of 300 units)
Combine yogurt, honey and lemon juice. open the vitamin E capsules and fold contents into the mix. Leave on skin for 15 minutes.

422. ALMOND-BUTTER HAND SOFTENER

1 T. almond oil
1 C. butter
Mix well. Before bed, massage mixture into

hands, then cover with white cotton gloves. Wear all night while sleeping.

423. Almond Cleanser

Grind almonds to a fine powder in a blender. Wet face then rub on almond powder. Rinse. Store powder in a tighly sealed container.

424. Amaze Body Mist

2 cups distilled water
3 tbs. vodka
5 drops hypericum perforatum essential oil
10 drops cypress essential oil
10 drops rosemary essential oil
Mix all the ingredients together in a spray bottle, shake well. Allow to settle for at least 12 hours. Store in a cool dry place.

425. AVOCADO-YOGURT HAND TREATMENT

1 mashed avocado Juice from 1/2 lemon 1/2 C. plain yogurt Petroleum jelly

Mix together the avocado, lemon juice and yogurt. Slather over hands; leave on for 10 to 15 minutes, then rinse off. This will gently slough off dull
skin and will gradually fade age spots, also. After rinsing, lavish on petroleum jelly or super-rich hand cream and then wear white cotton gloves for one hour or overnight for maximum hydrating.

Note: do not use this slougher more than twice a week as it can be irritating. Also, do not apply it to cuts or sores as it may sting.

426. Basic Skin Toner

Mix 1 cup witch hazel, 1/4 cup white vinegar and 1/4 tsp. mint
extract. If you want, drop in some fresh peppermint leaves. Dab on your face with a cotton ball to hydrate skin and remove excess dirt from pores. Cucumber A cooling, gentle astringent. Use the juice or mashed pulp.

427. Beeswax Lip Balm

2 tablespoons beeswax
1 tablespoon coconut oil
Melt the ingredients over a double boiler. Pour into a container while still hot since it will harden as it cools. Makes about 1/4 cup.

428. Blond Hair Highlighter

1/2 cup water
1/4 cup honey
1 tablespoon Irish moss

1/4 Cup molasses
Soak the Irish moss in the water for 5 minutes. Then simmer for several minutes over low heat until the mixture is thick. Add the remaining ingredients. Apply to freshly shampooed hair and let soak for 3-5 minutes. Then rinse off

with warm water. Makes about 1 cup, enough for two applications.

429. BLUEBERRY TONIC (soothes and nourishes skin)

Make this mask the day you plan to use it.
3 T. steamed, crushed blueberries
1/2 C. sour cream or plain yogurt
Purée ingredients in a blender at low speed until well mixed and fluffy. Apply to face and neck. Rinse off with tepid water after 15 to 20 minutes. If mask is too runny after blending, refrigerate for one hour.

430. BROWN SUGAR CALLUS EXFOLIATOR

1 C. brown sugar, moistened with rose water
1/2 C. petroleum jelly
Rub onto calluses on hands, knees and feet. Wash off.

431. Buttermilk and Fennel Cleansing Milk (For Oily Skin)

1/2 cup buttermilk
2 Tbsp crushed fennel seeds
Heat the milk and fennel seeds in top of double boiler for 30 minutes. Turn off heat, let steep for 2 hours. Strain, cool, pour into bottle and refrigerate. Keeps for 2 weeks.

432. CHAMOMILE STEAMING FACE CLEANSER

1 tsp. chamomile leaves
Mix in a heatproof bowl. Hold face 10 inches from water for 8 minutes; follow with a tightening mask.

433. Chamomile Cleansing Milk (For Dry and Sensitive Skin)

1/4 cup cream
1/4 cup milk
2 Tbsp chamomile flowers, fresh or dried
Simmer ingredients in top of a double boiler for about 30 minutes, do not allow milk to boil. Turn off heat and let sit for about 2 hours, strain. Keep refrigerated. Apply with cotton balls to the face. Variations: Use elderflowers, sweet violets or lime blossoms in place of chamomile. **434. Chamomile Baby Powder**
2 tbs. crumbled dried chamomile flowers
1/4 cup cornstarch
1 tbs. orrisroot
1/2 tsp. alum
Mix ingredients together in a bowl. Sift and store in powder shaker. Use to keep baby's skin soft and dry.

435. Chamomile / Mint Astringent (Non-alcoholic for Sensitive Skin)

1/2 cup chopped fresh mint (or 2 tbs. dried)
2 tbs. dried chamomile flowers, crushed
4 cups water
Combine ingredients in a small saucepan. Boil for 10 minutes, then remove

from heat and allow to steep for 5 minutes. Strain liquid into a jar, cover and refrigerate. Will keep 2 weeks refrigerated. Apply with cotton balls to skin. This astringent is especially good for sensitive or very oily skin.

436. Chocolate lip gloss

1 1/2 tsp grated cocoa butter
1/2 tsp coconut oil
1/8 tsp vitamin E oil
1/4 tsp grated chocolate or 3 small chcolate chips
In a double boiler or microwave heat the cocoa butter, coconut oil, and vitamin E oiluntil melted.

Stir in the chocolate chips and keep stirring until melted and well blended Pour into small container and allow to cool before using

437. CIDER STABILIZING RINSE

1/4 C. cider vinegar
1/4 C. water
Combine vinegar and water and gently wipe your face with the mixture. Let this rinse dry on your skin

438. Cinnamon Soap

Unscented glycerin soap
10 drops cinnamon oil
1 drop red food coloring (optional)
In a heavy saucepan, melt the glycerin soap

over low heat until liquefied. Remove the pan from the heat and stir in the cinnamon oil and food coloring until well mixed. Pour the soap into a mold and let set for 3 hours or until hardened. Makes one 4-ounce bar.

439. Citrus Astringent

3 tsp. lemon extract
Juice of one lime
1/2 cup rubbing alcohol
Combine ingredients in a small bowl. Transfer to a jar and shake well. Store in the refrigerator, will keep up to 6 months. Tightens pores, refreshes skin, and helps remove oils from skin.

440. Citrus Blooms Body Splash

2 cups distilled water
3 tbs. vodka
1 tbs. orange peel, finely chopped
1 tbs. lemon peel, finely chopped
5 drops lemon verbena essential oil
10 drops mandarin essential oil
10 drops orange essential oil
Combine the fruit peels with the vodka in a jar, cover and let stand for 1 week. Strain the liquid, add the essential oils and water to the liquid.
Let stand for 2 weeks, shaking jar once a day. Keep in a dark bottle or keep in a cool dark area.

441. Cocoa Butter Minty Lip Balm

1-1/2 parts cocoa butter 1-1/2 parts grated beeswax

3 parts edible vegetable oil of your choice (almond, apricot kernel, avocado, extra virgin olive, hemp seed, jojoba, kukui nut, macadamia nut, castor all work well... but keep in mind if you plan on selling lip balm or giving as a gift, that some people are allergic to nut oils)
Spearmint and/or peppermint flavoring oil
Melt the cocoa butter and beeswax slowly and carefully in a microwave, or over a double boiler on the stove until melted. Add oil and stir well. Add spearmint or peppermint flavoring oils, or both, a few drops at a time, to taste. Gently reheat if needed. Cool slightly before pouring into
containers. To test consistency, place a drop on a spoon and set in the refrigerator to cool for a few minutes. Test on your lips. For a softer lip balm, add more oil. For a harder lip balm, add more beeswax.

442. Cooling Foot and Body Powder

1/2 cup powdered arrowroot
1/2 cup cosmetic clay
2 tbs. powdered ginger
20 drops tea tree oil (or lavender essential oil)
This light, fragrant powder absorbs moisture and fights bacteria to eradicate perspiration and

body odor. It also helps relieve athlete's foot. It contains tea tree oil and powdered ginger, both of which have antiseptic and antifungal action. If you're making a body powder, you may prefer to use lavender essential oil in place of the tea tree oil; it has a little

less antiseptic power, but more fragrance. Instructions for making powder: In a large jar, combine the arrowroot, cosmetic clay and ginger. Cover and shake to mix. Add the tea tree or lavender oil and shake again. You may want to sift the powder through a fine mesh strainer to break up any drops of oil. Store in a covered, dark glass jar. Apply as needed to feet or

body. Stored in a cool, dry place, the powder will keep indefinitely.

443. Cooling Summer Body Spray

1 tbs. witch hazel
1 tsp. lemon extract
1 tsp. cucumber extract
1 cup water
For a refreshing cool feeling, make an after shower spray by combining all the ingredients. Place in a pump spay bottle and spritz onto skin.

444. Cornmeal Cleanser (for Oily Skin)

Castile soap
1 Tsp Cornmeal

Wet face. Pour a little castile soap into the palm of your hand, add cornmeal. Mix meal and soap into a lather, wash face, being careful to avoid the delicate skin around the eyes.

445. CUCUMBER-LEMON TONIC (soothing astringent for oily skin)

This tightens pores, soothes sunburn, and can be used as a natural deodorant, also.
1 C. witch hazel
Juice of 1 lemon

3 T. coarsely chopped cucumber
Mix in a clean glass bottle, then let set for 2 days. Remove cucumber. Keep lotion in a cool place or the refrigerator to use as a splash.

446. CUCUMBER-ROSE REFRESHER

3 oz. cucumber juice
3 oz. distilled witch hazel
1 1/2 oz. rose water
Mix together and place in a clean jar. Refrigerate. After cleansing face, soak a clean cotton ball with the lotion and gently pat over skin.

447. Custom - Scented Glycerin Soap

1 lb. block of glycerin soap
1/8 to 1/4 oz. of essential fragrance oil
1 cup boiling water and 1/2 cup powdered herbs or rose petals or oatmeal, cornmeal or almond meal (herbs & meals are optional)...

OR... 1/4 to 1/2 cup herbal infusion (tea)
Melt glycerin in double boiler with water (or herbal infusion). If using powders, stir in with non-metallic spoon. Let cool slightly (not enough to harden - still pourable) and add the scent. Mix in and pour into molds or saran wrap-lined box. Let harden, cut into bars and bevel the edges and rough spots with a paring knife. This recipe can also be made with castile soap flakes or they can be used in combination with the glycerin soap.

448. Custom - Scented Hair Gel

2 tbs. flax seeds
1 cup water
Few drops essential oils
Place flax seeds and water in a saucepan and bring to a boil. Remove from heat and let sit for about 15 to 20 minutes. Strain and allow to cool completely. Add the essential oils when cooled. Place in a glass container and store at room temperature.

449. Custom - Scented Liquid / Gel Soap

2 cups soap flakes or grated bar soap
1/2 gallon water
2 tbs. glycerin
Fragranced or essential oil of your choice
Food coloring of your choice (optional)
Mix first 3 ingredients together in a large pot or dutch oven. Set over low heat, stirring

occasionally, until the soap has dissolved. Add fragrance

oil and food coloring and mix well. Transfer to a jar and cover tightly. For a less thick gel soap, use 1 gallon of water.

450. Do it Yourself "Petroleum" Jelly

2 oz. beeswax or wax of your choice.
1 cup of the oil of your choice.
Melt the beeswax in a double boiler or in microwave. Stir in the oil Remove the mixture from the heat and stir until it is cool.

451. Eggwhite Toner

Clean face thoroughly using any natural cleanser. Apply raw eggwhites to the skin and leave on for at least 15 minutes. Wash off with tepid

water .

452. EGG-HONEY MOISTURIZER

1 egg yolk
2 T. honey
Mix ingredients together until a light paste is formed; apply to face and neck, avoiding eye area and mouth. Leave on for 10 to 15 minutes; rinse off thoroughly with tepid water.

453. Enchanted Body Mist

2 cups distilled water
3 tbs. vodka
5 drops everlasting essential oil
10 drops peony essential oil
10 drops sandalwood essential oil
Mix all the ingredients together in a spray
bottle, shake well. Allow to settle for at least 12
hours. Store in a cool dry place.

454. Frizz Tamer for Hair

1/2 cup conditioner
1/4 cup honey
1 tbs. almond oil
Mix ingredients well. Pour mixture over damp
hair, work it in. Leave it on for about 20
minutes for a good deep conditioning. Wash
out. This works for all hair types.

455. FRUIT PUNCH REFRESHER

1/2 C. lemon yogurt
1 tsp. lemon juice
1 tsp. lime juice
1 tsp. grapefruit juice
Mix; leave on face for 10 minutes. Rinse with
cold club soda.

456. Hair Color - Blonde Highlights for Hair

1 cup lemon juice
3 cups chamomile tea (brewed and then
cooled)
Mix ingredients together. Pour over damp hair.

Let it sit for 1 hour while you sit in the sun.
Wash out.

457. Hair Color - Red Highlights for Hair

1/2 cup beet juice
1/2 cup carrot juice
Mix ingredients together. Pour over damp hair.
Let it sit for 1 hour while you sit in the sun.
Wash out.

458. Herbal Aftershave

1/2 cup rubbing alcohol
1/4 cup witch hazel
1/2 cup distilled water
3 drops oil of benzoin
1 tbs. olive oil
1/2 cup dried herbs and/or a few drops of
essential oils of your preference (some ideas for
herbs: rosemary, sage, cinnamon, cloves,
crushed lavender flowers, orange or lemon
peels, etc.)

Combine ingredients in a jar. Cover and place in
a dark, fairly cool place. Shake the jar once or
twice a day for 2 to 3 days. Strain out herbs
and refrigerate.

459. Herbal Blemish Treatment

1 cup water
1/4 C parsley
1 TBSP mint leaves
1/4 watercress
3 medium size carrots(peeled and xhopped)

1 egg white
Bring first 4 ingredients to a boil, reduce heat
and simmer for 30 minutes. Remove from heat
and let cool. In a blender mix infusion with
carrots and egg whiteon medium speed for 45
seconds
Apply to face , let sit for 10 to 20 minutes.
Rinse off with warm water Cover and refrigerate
immediately, discard after 3 days

460. HERB GARDEN SPLASH

2 C. white vinegar 1/4 C. honey
1 tsp. sage
1 tsp. thyme

1 tsp. savory
1 tsp. ground cloves
1 tsp. crushed bay leaves
Combine all ingredients and store in a sterilized
glass jar for 1 week. Shake occasionally to mix
contents. Strain and pour into a tightly capped
bottle.

461. HERBAL FACE STEAM (deep pore cleanser)

1 qt. water
1 handful any herbs*
Juice and peel of 1/2 lemon
Bring water to a boil. Add juice and peel of
lemon and herbs. Turn off the heat and take the
pot to a table. Cover your hair with a shower
cap or towel and drape another towel over your

head and the pot, holding your face about 10 inches above the water. Keep your eyes closed and let the steam do its magic cleansing for about 15 minutes. Afterward, rinse with COLD water to close the pores.
* Use any herbs you have available: rosemary, thyme, mint, marjoram, basil, parsley, cloves, caraway, anise or fennel seeds, chamomile, lavender or
elder flowers.

462. High Protein Moisturizer

Beat 1 egg yolk into 1 cup whole milk. Apply to face with fingertips. Bottle and store remainder in refrigerator

463. Honey Hand Cleanser

2 tablespoons honey
1 tablespoon liquid soap
1/4 cup almond or walnut oil
Combine the ingredients and mix until smooth. Makes about 1/3 cup.

464. Honey Cleanser (For Dry Skin)

Castile soap
1 Tsp Honey
Wet face. Pour a little castile soap into the palm of your hand, add honey. Mix honey and soap into a lather, wash face.

465. Hot Oil Treatment for Hair

1 tsp. soybean oil
2 tsp. castor oil
Few drops fragrance oil (optional)
Combine ingredients and warm on low heat.
Massage mixture into the scalp and hair. Wrap
hair in a hot towel for 15 minutes. Shampoo
and rinse out.

466. Lemon Toner

1/2 cup lemon juice
1 cup distilled water
2/3 cup witch hazel
Combine all ingredients. Pour into a clean bottle
or decorative
cosmetics container. Shake well before using.
Apply with a clean cotton ball. Note: Lemon is a
strong astringent, dilute with water before
using, being careful to keep away from eyes.

467. LEMON ASTRINGENT (for oily skin)

1/2 C. witch hazel
1/4 C. lemon juice
Mix. Apply to face and neck with a clean cotton
ball.

468. LEMON RINSE

This is the strongest acid rinse. Mix a fresh
batch every five days. It becomes stale after
the fifth day and should be discarded.
1/4 C. lemon juice, freshly-squeezed
1 1/2 C. water

Combine lemon juice and water. After cleansing, smooth mixture over your face and allow to air dry.

469. LEMON SOAK (for dry, rough feet)

1 bowl warm water
Juice of 1 lemon
Add lemon juice to warm water in bowl. Soak feet for 15 to 20 minutes.

470. Lemony Lavender Toner

3 drops lemon oil
3 drops lavender oil
3 teaspons of distilled water
Use a soft cotton ball to massage mixture into the skin after
cleansing. Follow with a moisturizer if desired

471. LUSCIOUS BODY POLISHER

2 C. plain yogurt
1 T. wheat germ
1 T. honey
1 T. almond oil*
* Omit almond oil if skin is acne-prone.
Mix all ingredients. Dampen skin in shower and massage mixture all over.

Rinse with warm water. Rinse immediately with cold water to boost circulation.

472. Makeup Remover and Moisturizer

1/2 cup paraffin
1 cup mineral oil

1/2 cup water
2 tbs. alum
Slowly heat paraffin with the oil in a double
boiler. In a separate saucepan, heat the water
until it simmers, then dissolve the alum in it.
Let cook, then add to the warm mineral oil and
paraffin mixture. As everything cools, the
paraffin will rise to the top. Drain off the water.
The residue is your makeup remover.

473. Margarine

Buy a pound of natural margarine from the
health food store, NOT the supermarket. Store
in refrigerator. Apply enough to cover smooth
skin. It will absorb into the skin and
surprisingly, does not leave a greasy residue.

474. Mechanic's Hand Cleanser

1 cup borax
1 to 2 tsp. pure turpentine
1 tsp. sweet orange essential oil
1 cup ground soap
With very clean hands, work the turpentine and
essential oil into the borax until there are no
lumps left, then work into the soap. Keep it in a
wide-mouthed jar or tin that's easy for him to
open when his hands are greasy, and which you
won't mind getting dirty on the outside. Don't
forget to put a nail brush and pumice stone out
with the hand cleanser.

475. Misty Passions Perfume

3 drops passionflower oil
2 drops ylang-ylang oil
3 drops neroli oil
1/2 pint (300ml) 70 percent alcohol or vodka
Pour the alcohol into a bottle or jar. Add the oils
and shake well. Let stand for 1 week before
using.

476. Milk and Honey Cleanser

Mix 1 tsp warm honey with 1 tablespoon milk or
cream. This recipe should be prepared fresh
each time.

477. MOLDED MASSAGE OIL BAR

4 T. solid vegetable shortening 3 T. solid cocoa
butter
2 T. solid coconut oil
1 T. beeswax

1 T. paraffin wax
10 drops orange essential oil (or whatever you
like)
Heat all the above, except essential oil, in a
microwave (power 7) for approximately 3
minutes or melt in a double boiler.
Stir until liquid. If you want them colored, add
a crayon or wax dye. Beat

for several minutes until emulsified and slightly
thick. If it isn't
thickening, place your bowl in ice water as you
beat it with an electric mixer.Add essential
oil.Pour into metal or lightly oiled plastic/glass

molds.(Chocolate molds work well and are about the right amount for a body massage.) Refrigerate until set.Wrap in plastic and store in a cool place.

To use, simply hand warm your molded oil and give a massage to your favorite person or give yourself a foot massage.

478. NATURAL LEMON SKIN EXFOLIANT

1/2 to 2/3 C. granulated sugar
Juice of 1 lemon
Mix sugar and lemon juice to form a paste. While showering invigorate your skin with the paste. Use the inside of the lemon rind to rub heels and elbows.

479. Oriental Nights Perfume

4 drops sandalwood 4 drops musk
3 drops frankincense 2 tsp. jojoba oil

Mix all the ingredients together and shake well. Allow perfume to settle for at least 12 hours. Store in a cool dry place.

480. Paraffin Wax Treatment For Hands -

You will need:
1 block paraffin wax (about 4 oz)
an ounce of oil
20 drops of essential oil... lavender is rather nice

189 of
a few drops of olive oil (you will use this to coat your hands)
a casserole dish that you have greased with oil before hand
plastic sandwich bags
Melt the paraffin, the ounce of oil, the scented oil in a double
boiler. Be sure to use a double boiler for safety purposes. Very
carefully pour the wax into the dish and wait until a skin has
formed on the top of the wax. When this happens, the temperature should be about right for submerging your hands.**But before you do, be sure to test the wax for comfort in case the wax is still a
little too warm for your liking. Testing a little on your wrist
usually works. Get your hands ready by washing them and then pat them dry with paper towel. Smooth on the olive oil and be sure
to cover every inch of your hands and fingers. Dip each hand into
the wax repeatedly until you have several layers of wax built up on
your hands. Have someone help you put on the sandwich bags onto each hand and then relax for about 30 minutes. For added benefit, place a bath towel over your hands as you wait. This is a perfect time to
watch a half hour of tv. Now comes the time to

remove the wax... simply peel it away. Start at the wrist area and pull it down. It should come off in large sections. Give yourself a little hand massage and
you are done.

481. Protein Toner

Beat together 1 Tbsp milk, 1 tsp honey and 1 egg. Apply to face and
neck. Leave on as long as desired. Rinse off with warm water followed by a splash of cold.

482. Rose

Use 2 parts rose water and 1 part glycerin to make a lotion. Apply nightly and work into skin.

483. ROSE WATER

1 C. rose petals
1/2 C. rubbing alcohol
1 1/2 C. water
Simmer rose petals in water for 10 minutes. Strain. Preserve with alcohol or just refrigerate without preserving. Store up to 1 week in the refrigerator.

484. Rose Water & Glycerine Astringent

1/2 pint olive oil
1 ounce rose water
a few drops of glycerin 1 ounce vodka

485. ROSE-ROSEMARY LOTION

1 oz. rose petal tea or rose water
1 oz. rosemary tea
1 T. egg white

Whirl in the blender. Store in a clean, tightly-capped, jar in the refrigerator.

486. Sage Astringent

4 Tbsp dried sage
4 Tbsp vodka
1/4 tsp borax
3 Tbsp witch hazel
10 drops glycerin or honey
Steep the sage in vodka for 2 weeks then strain. Dissolve borax in witch hazel, stir in the saged vodka and glycerin. Pour into bottle with a tight cap. Shake before each use.

487. Sesame Oil Cleanser (For Dry Skin)

Apply sesame oil to face and neck. Remove oil and makeup with a washcloth that has been soaked in hot water and wrung out. Finish with a rinse
of the pH Balancer.

488. Scented Rocks (A Nice Alternative to Potpourri)

1/2 cup plain flour
1/2 cup salt
1/4 tsp. essential oil in your favorite scent
2/3 cups boiling water
Food coloring, if desired

In bowl, mix dry ingredients well. Add essential oil and boiling water to

dry ingredients. (Scent will be strong, but will fade slightly when dry.) For colored stones, blend in food coloring, one drop at a time, until desired shade is reached. Blend ingredients and form balls. Allow stones to dry. Place rocks in a bowl or dish to scent a room.

489. SKIN BOOSTER

4 T. dried dandelions
4 T. chamomile
5 T. rosemary
1 (12-inch) square muslin or cotton
Place herbs in center of fabric. Bunch edges of fabric together. Secure with rubber band or string to form a scrubber. Place in a pot of boiling water. Remove from stove. Steep 10 minutes. Remove scrubber and save the water as

it contains herbal juices. Place scrubber in a glass dish until it cools to
room temperature. Sweep over entire body, one area at a time, with long strokes, continually moistening scrubber in the herbal water. First stroke
in an up-and-down direction, then in a circular motion. Leave herbal residue on for 20 minutes; rinse with tepid water.

490. SKIN CONDITIONER (for oily or scaly skin)

1 oz. lemongrass
1 oz. cornmeal
1 oz. witch hazel
1 oz. rose petals
Blend lemongrass, cornmeal, witch hazel and rose petals, then mix 1 ounce of this mixture with 1 quart boiling water. Let steep 20 minutes. Strain into

bath water. Soak at least 10 minutes. Use two times a week or more.

491. "Smelly Jelly" Air Fresheners

1/4 to 1/2 cup AGROSOKE polymer crystals (sold at Walmart, Lowe's, Home Depot, etc...)
Clean water (distilled, bottled or from a water filter)
Food coloring

HIGH QUALITY fragrance oil (that's the key)
Jelly jars and ring tops (Mason makes nice quilted-looking ones in 3
sizes - perfect)
Pretty lace fabric OR very loose-weave fabric cut into squares (4" x 4" or a little larger)
Get a large bowl or pot and put the 1/4 to 1/2 cup of crystals in it. Fill
it up 3/4 full with hot water and a few drops of food coloring. Remember - these crystals expand a few hundred times their original size,

so pick a bowl large enough! Stir the colored mixture to saturate all the crystals. Wait. Every 10 minutes or so give the crystals a stir. After about 30 minutes all the water should be gone and the crystals should be gel-like. I f not, wait some more. It will absorb all the colored water. Next, you can add the fragrance oil to the whole bowl of gel OR you can split it up into separate bowls and scent them separately. You only need a few tablespoons of scent. After you add the fragrance oil, stir well. I make it rather strong so it never runs out of scent.
Line up the jelly jars, fabric squares and jar top rings. Add the jelly to
the jars almost to the top. Place a fabric square over the top. Screw the jar top ring on to secure the fabric in place. Then pour a tablespoon of

water through the fabric top. Do not let the water come out the top. Fill almost to the top only.
Lastly, tie a ribbon around the ring if you want to or just leave it as it
is. Don't throw away the jar top circles! These are great to use when you don't want to use the smelly jelly right away. Just put these on the jars BEFORE the fabric is added, to seal in the scent. Then take them off and reapply the fabric and rings when you're ready to use your smelly jelly. These last for months, but remember - water must be poured through the fabric top every week or so to keep them from

drying out - very important!! If you happen to forget, they can be brought back from total dry out though.

I forgot one and had nothing but crystals and oil in the jar, but I added some water... a few hours later, a perfect smelly jelly!

492. Soapless Hand Cleanser

2 tablespoons honey
2 tablespoons vegetable oil
1 tablespoon oatmeal or ground almonds
1 tablespoon glycerin
2 tablespoons witch hazel
Combine the ingredients and mix until smooth. This may be used to remove dirt from the hands and fingernails, and is less drying on the skin than
soap and water. Makes enough for 1 application.

493. SOOTHING CUCUMBER CREAM

1 whole cucumber, unpeeled
1/2 oz. white paraffin
2 oz. sweet almond oil
Cut the cucumber into chunks and purée it in the food processor or blender. Strain the pulp through a strainer lined with cheesecloth.

Melt the wax in a small bowl in the top of a glass or enamel double boiler over medium heat. As soon as the wax is melted, slowly add the oil, stirring gently. Add strained cucumber and blend thoroughly.

Remove the pot from the heat and cover with a clean towel. Let the mixture cool very slowly to prevent crystals from forming in the wax. Stir mixture once or twice until cool. When the mixture is completely cool and smooth, store it in a tightly capped glass container in the refrigerator. It will keep for two months.

To use, smooth a bit of cream every night around the tender skin of your face and neck.

494. Soothing Scented Aftershave

2 cups rubbing alcohol
1 tbs. glycerin
1 tbs. dried lavender
1 tsp. dried rosemary
1 tsp. ground cloves

Stir ingredients together in a bowl. Transfer to a jar, cover, and refrigerate for 3 to 4 days. Shake occasionally to mix ingredients. After 3 to 4 days, strain out herbs. Keep refrigerated, will keep for 1 to 2 months. Yield: 2 cups.

495. Strawberry

Mash strawberries, use as an astringent and cleansing face mask.

Sweet Butter Cleansing Cream (For Dry Skin)
Whip sweet, unsalted butter, transfer to container with a tid lid. May be stored at room temperature away from heat sources or refrigerate.

496. STRAWBERRIES AND CREAM ASTRINGENT (for oily or blemished skin)

1 handful strawberries
1 heaping T. heavy cream

Mash strawberries by hand or in a blender. Add heavy cream and mix well. Spread thickly on face and neck (a shaving brush is handy for this) and let your skin benefit for 10 minutes. Tissue off, then splash face and neck with cool water.

497. STRAWBERRY TONER (oily skin astringent)

1/2 C. mashed strawberries
1/2 C. sour cream or plain yogurt
Purée ingredients in a blender at low speed until sell mixed and fluffy. Apply to face and neck; rinse with tepid water after 30 minutes. If mask is too runny after blending, refrigerate for one hour. Make mask the day you plan to use it.

498. SUPER DRY SKIN FORMULA

1 pt. pure aloe gel
1 oz. (tube) zinc oxide paste
2 T. sunflower oil
Few drops vitamin E oil
Whip ingredients together. Store in a container. Smooth over damp skin after
a shower or bath.

499. Swimming pool hair care- to keep blonde

hair from turning green
2 TBSP baking soda
1/4 C lemon juice
1 tsp mild shampoo
Mix together all ingredients until well blended. Wet hair and massage mixture well into hair and scalp, making sure hair ends are coated. Cover hair with plastic bag or shower cap and leave on 30

minutes. Rinse hair well and shampoo as usual.

500. Violet

Simmer violet flowers in a little milk to make a softening and mildly astringent face lotion.

501. VINEGAR FACIAL CONDITIONER (for moderately oily skin)

1 C. water
1 T. vinegar (any type)
Mix water and vinegar in a bottle. Apply up to 1/4 teaspoon of mixture to face after each cleansing. Let dry naturally, without patting.

502. VINEGAR RINSE

1/4 C. apple cider vinegar
1 basin warm water
This restores the natural pH balance or acid mantle to your skin.

Pour vinegar into warm water. Splash your face thoroughly. Let dry without using a towel. Acne sufferers should try this also, but be sure to start
with a perfectly clean face.

503. Whispering Rain Body Mist

2 cups distilled water
3 tbs. vodka
5 drops sandalwood essential oil
10 drops bergamot essential oil
10 drops cassis essential oil
Mix all the ingredients together in a spray bottle, shake well. Allow to settle for at least 12 hours. Store in a cool dry place.

504. WITCH HAZEL SKIN CLARIFIER

3/4 C. witch hazel
1/4 C. rubbing alcohol
Mix the ingredients and store in a tightly capped, sterilized glass bottle. To use, moisten a clean cotton ball and clean your face with this solution after washing and before applying moisturizer. Your skin should feel tingly while using this clarifier.

Tooth and Mouth Care

All Natural Toothpaste

Ingredients:
1/4 tsp peppermint oil
1/4 tsp spearmint

1/4 cup arrowroot
1/4 cup powdered orrisroot
1/4 cup water
1 tsp ground sage
Instructions:
Mix all of the dry ingredients in a bowl. Add water until the paste is desired the consistency. Store at room temperature in a tightly covered jar.
You can also substitute 1/2 tsp each of oil of cinnamon and oil of cloves for peppermint/ spearmint if desired.

Breath Fresheners

1) Chew fresh parsley to sweeten the breath.
2) Chew fennel seeds to freshen the breath.
3) Chew anise seeds to freshen the breath.
4) Chew a few peppermint or spearmint leaves or drink a cup of peppermint tea 5) Add 1 drop of myrrh oil to 1 cup of cooled, boiled water. Use as gargle/mouthwash. tea

Old Fashioned Tooth Powder

2 Tbsp dried lemon or orange rind
1/4 cup baking soda
2 Tsp salt
Place rinds in food processor, grind until peel becomes a fine powder. Add baking

soda and salt then process a few seconds more until you have a fine powder. Store in an airtight tin or jar. Dip moistened toothbrush into mixture, brush as usual.

Basic Toothpaste

1 Tsp of the Old Fashioned Tooth Powder 1/4 Tsp Hydrogen peroxide
Mix into a paste and brush as usual.

Loretta's Toothpaste

1 Tsp baking soda,
1/4 Tsp hydrogen peroxide
1 drop oil of peppermint
Mix to make a paste, dip toothbrush into mixture, brush as usual.

Lemon Clove Tooth Cleanser

Mix:
Small amount of finely powdered sage
1 ounce of finely powdered myrrh
1 pound powdered arrow root
3 ounces powdered orris root
20 drops oil of lemon
10 drops oil of cloves
12 drops oil of bergamot
Rub oils into the powdered ingredients until thoroughly mixed.

Strawberry Tooth Cleanser

1 Tsp of the above Old Fashioned Tooth Powder
1 Tbsp crushed ripe strawberries

Mix strawberries and powder into a paste and brush as usual.

Vanilla & Rose Geranium Toothpaste

1/2 ounce powdered chalk
3 ounces powdered orris root
4 teaspoons of tincture of vanilla
15 drops oil of rose geranium
Honey, enough to make a paste
Combine all ingredients and mix until you have a paste the consistency you like. Store in an airtight container.
Use a clean stick (popsicle) to scoop paste onto brush. Store the stick in same container.

Tooth Care

1) Mash some fresh strawberries and use as you would any other "tooth paste" 2) Using fresh sage leaves, rub over the teeth to clean and whiten.

Rosemary-Mint Mouthwash

2 1/2 cups distilled or mineral water 1 tsp fresh mint leaves
1tsp rosemary leaves
1 tsp anise seeds

Boil the water, add herbs and seeds, infuse for 20 minutes. Cool, strain and use as a gargle/ mouthwash. If you wish to make up a larger quantity, double or triple the recipe then add 1 tsp of tincture of myrrh as a natural preservative.

Spearmint Mouthwash

6 ounces water
2 ounces vodka
4 teaspoons liquid glycerine
1 teaspoon aloe vera gel
10-15 drops Spearmint essential oil
Boil water and vodka, add glycerine and aloe vera gel. Remove from the heat, let cool slightly. Add spearmint oil, shake well. Pour into bottle, cap tightly.

Nail & Hand Care

For dry nails

2 tsp. gelatin
1/2 glass fruit juice
mix together, drink at once
repeat daily for atleast 6 weeks. Regularly, soak fingernails in a bowl of warmed olive oil for about 5 min. Dry with soft towel, gently pushing back cuticles.

Dill And Horsetail Nail Bath

2 tb (30ml) chopped horsetail
2 tb (30ml) dill seed
1 c (225ml) boiling water
Pour the water over the two herbs and steep for at least an hour.
Strain the liquid into a bottle. Both these herbs

contain silicic acid, which helps to strengthen nails. Warm the mixture before using and soak your nails in it for ten minutes every other day.

For weak nails

Massage wheat germ oil into cuticles.

Fingernail Treatments

1) Beat 1 egg yolk in a small bowl. Soak fingernails for 5 minutes. Rinse.
2) Forget the Palmolive Madge! Make a solution of pure castile soap and water in a large bowl, soak hands and nails for about 10-15 minutes.

Dill & Horsetail Nail Soak

2 Tbsp chopped horsetail herb
2 Tbsp dill seeds
1 cup boiling water
Pour water over herbs, steep for 1-2 hours. Strain and bottle. To use: warm some of the solution, pour into a small bowl, soak nails for 10 minutes.

Lady's Mantle Hand Mask

2 Tbsp finely ground oatmeal 1Tbsp lady's mantle infusion 1 tsp avocado oil
1 tsp lemon juice

1 tsp glycerin
Mix all to form a smooth paste. Apply to hands at bedtime. Leave on for 1/2 hour, wash off and

apply moisturizing cream overnight (wear gloves) Wash off in the morning.

Cornmeal Hands Mask

Mix 1/4 cup corn meal with 3 Tbsp. milk. Heat over low heat until a paste forms. Add 1 drop almond oil. Let cool. Spread on hands, leave on for about 10 minutes. Rinse.

Lady's Mantle Hand Lotion

2 Tbsp of a strong infusion of lady's mantle
2 Tbsp glycerin
2 tsp carrageen moss (Irish Moss) melted in a little hot water
4 Tbsp vodka
10 drops essential oil of rose or geranium
Stir glycerin into melted moss. Add essential oil to vodka, then blend into the glycerin mixture. Stir in lady's mantle infusion, blend well. Pour into jar, cap tightly. Shake before using.

Heavy Duty Barrier Cream

4 Tbsp Unpetroleum Jelly (available in natural foods stores)
2 handfuls fresh elderflowers
Melt jelly, add elderflowers. Steep for 45 minutes, reheating the jelly when it solidifies. Reheat until mixture is liquified, strain through a fine sieve into a jar. Cool, then cap tightly.

Heavy Duty Gardeners Hand Cream

2 Tablespoons of shaved beeswax 1/2 Teaspoon
of carnuba wax
2 Tablespoons of jojoba oil
1 Teaspoon of aloe vera gel

10 drops of Vitamin E oil (or 4 capsules)
1 drop of your favorite essentail oil for
fragrance
Melt the first four ingredients in a stainless
steel pot on the stove or use a glass pyrex cup
in the microwave. Remove from heat and beat
until cool, adding the Vitamin E oil before
mixture thickens. Continue beating until this
mixture becomes creamy. Add your favorite
essential oil, continue beating until cream has
completely cooled. Spoon your cream into a jar,
store in a cool dark place.

Banana Hand & Foot Cream

Dry hands and feet will become smooth and
soft overnight if you mix: Bananas
Honey
Lemon juice

Natural margarine
Smear on hands and wear white gloves to bed.
Wash off in the morning. For dry feet, smear
the mixture on and wear heavy socks to bed,
wash off in the morning.

Wheatgerm Hot Oil Fingernail Treatment

Soak fingernails in warmed wheat germ oil for about 5 minutes. Wipe off oil, then massage nails. Strengthens weak and brittle nails.

Eye Care

1) The best overall eye tonic is eyebright (an herb). Make a tea of it and either use the teabags or soak cotton balls or soft gauze in the tea and apply to eyes as a compress while lying down.

2) For puffy and swollen eyes, make a wet compress of 4 Tbsp. freshly grated raw potato. Place on the eyes for about 15 minutes, then rinse with cold water.
3) To reduce swelling and for bags under the eyes, brew a cup of strong rosehip tea. Soak 2 cotton balls in the tea or use 2 tea bags, lie down and place over the eyes. 4) For dark cirles, cut a fresh fig in half, place a half over each eye.

5) To soothe tired, irritated eyes, cut the end of a cumber into 1/4 in thick slices. Apply a cool slice to each eye.
6) Raw potato slices laid on sore eyes reduces heat and redness.
7) For eye puffiness, any tea bag (herbal is better, especially eyebright), slightly cooled, placed on the eyes while you rest.

8) For tired or bloodshot eyes, soak sterile cotton balls or soft cloth in cold skim milk.

Place over eyes for 10 minutes. Rinse entire face in warm,then cool, water.
9) To lighten dark circles under your eyes, wrap a grated raw potato in cheesecloth and apply to eyelids for 15-20 minutes. Rinse with warm water.

Lip Balm and Lip Gloss

Here's How to Make Your Own Lip Balm and Lip Gloss! 1.) The basic formula is:

1/4 cup vegetable or nut oil
1/4 ounce beeswax
1 teaspoon honey or glycerine (humectants)
1/2 to 1 teaspoon natural flavoring oil aka Essential Oil.

Heat the oil and beeswax in a double boiler (or microvave) until the beeswax is melted.
Remove from heat and whip with an electric beater until creamy.
Add the honey or glycerine and approx 5 drops flavoring oil; whip some more. Add more flavoring if desired. Store in small glass jars, small tupperware bowls, decorative tins or film containers. Try different oils on your lips to choose the best one for your skin and taste preference. If the Balm is too hard (waxy), add more oil to your mixture. If it is too soft, add more wax.

You can add a few drops of beet juice for a beautiful & natural red color.

But instead of going to that trouble, you can just shave off a little of your lip stick for that beautiful (not natural) color. Don't use food coloring, it may contain alcohol base.

Never use extracts found in cooking sections of the grocery stores as they contain alcohol. Use safe essential oils. The good part about them is they have thousands of great flavors. Comfrey, Rosemary, Tea Tree or Camphor Oils are excellent for healing effects.

How do you know if it's time to throw away your gloss? If it changes color, odor, or texture, throw it away.

Basic Lip Gloss ? Fun!

Ingredients: Paraffin wax Coconut oil Petroleum jelly

Candy melts (to color the gloss and make it taste sweet) Oil-based candy flavoring (if you want a special flavor) Grater
Wax paper

Ziploc bag

Small container (recycle old lip gloss / balm containers or other makeup containers, even 35mm film containers work well. Other places to look include, stores that carry beads, crafts, or fishing tackle supplies.

How to:
Grate a bit of paraffin wax onto wax paper. Put 1/4 teaspoon grated wax into the plastic bag. Add 1 teaspoon coconut oil, 1 teaspoon petroleum jelly, and 1 candy melt to color the gloss and make it sweet. Add 1/8 teaspoon oil-based candy flavoring if you like. Seal the bag and put it in a bowl of hot water to melt the ingredients, for approximately 3-5 minutes. (Use tap water! Please never use a microwave or stove to heat the water). When all the ingredients are melted, take the bag out of the water. Move the ingredients around in bag to mix. Make sure you work quickly. Clip off a tiny corner of the bag and squeeze gloss into the clean container. Let it set for an hour. If you can't wait that long, just put this in the refrigerator for 15 minutes. Use a cotton swab to apply gloss to help your product last longer. Your lip-gloss should last a long time. If it changes color, odor, or texture, though, throw it away.

2.) Basic Lip Balm II

1/2 ounce beeswax beads, refined
4 ounces sweet almond oil
2 teaspoons essential oil or food flavoring oil

Put the 4 ounces of sweet almond oil in measuring cup, add beeswax beads and melt in microwave. Stir with spoon, and when cooled a bit, add essential or flavoring oil. Pour into jars or containers.

3.) Cranberry Lip Gloss

1 tablespoon sweet almond oil 10 fresh cranberries
1 teaspoon honey
1 drop of vitamin E oil

Mix all the ingredients together in a microwave-safe bowl.
Microwave for a couple of minutes or until the mixture just begins to boil.
(Bowl may also be heated in a pan of water on a stovetop).
Stir well and gently crush the berries.
Cool mixture for five minutes and then strain through a fine sieve to remove all the fruit pieces. Stir again and set aside to cool completely.
When cool, transfer into a small portable plastic container or tin.

4.)Silky Smooth Lip Balm

2 Teaspoons Olive Oil
1/2 Teaspoon Grated Beeswax or Beeswax Pellets 1/2 Teaspoon Shea Butter or Cocoa Butter

1/2 Teaspoon Honey
Any Flavored Oil To Taste
1 Vitamin E Capsule (as a preservative) (optional)

5.) Honey Balm

3 oz. Almond Oil
2 Teaspoons Honey
1/2 oz. Beeswax or Beeswax Pellets
1 Vitamin E Capsule (as a preservative) 1-4
Drops Essential Oil

6.) Almond Lip Gloss

2 Teaspoons Grated Beeswax or Beeswax
Pellets 3 - 6 Drops Flavored Oil
1 Teaspoon Sweet Almond Oil
3 Drops Honey

1 1/2 Teaspoon Cocoa Butter
1 Vitamin E Capsule (as a preservative)

7.) Helps heal cold sores.

1 oz. Emu Oil
1 oz. Almond Oil
1 oz. Avocado Oil
1/2 oz. Shaved Beeswax or Beeswax Pellets 1/4
oz. Aloe Vera Gel
6 Drops Lavender Essential Oil
2 Drops Tea Tree Essential Oil
3 Drops Lime Essential Oil

8. Honey Lip Balm

2 tsp. olive oil
1/2 tsp. beeswax
1/2 tsp. cocoa butter
1/2 tsp. honey
3 drops essential oil (I like orange.) 1 vitamin E
capsule

Measure oil, beeswax and cocoa butter into a glass or enamel pan.
Melt over low heat. A hotplate works well and reduces the risk of overheating the oils. Stir the mixture often until the wax is melted. Remove from heat and stir in the honey and essential oil. Pinch open the vitamin E capsule and squeeze the contents into the mixture. Stir well. Pour the mixture into containers.

9.) Aloe Vera Lip Gloss

1 tsp aloe vera gel 1/2 tsp coconut oil
1 tsp petroleum jelly

Mix the ingredients in a glass bowl, and microwave for 1 - 2 minutes. Pour into container.

10.) Vasoline Lip Balm

3 parts vasoline 1 part beeswax flavoring

Mix well

11.) Chocolate Balm

3 Tbsp. Cocoa Butter
4-5 Chocolate Chips
1 capsule, Vitamin E
Melt and blend ingredients with a spoon until smooth, put into a container and refrigerate until solid.

12.) Vanilla Lip Gloss

1 tablespoon grates beeswax 1/2 tablespoon coconut oil 1/8 teaspoon vitamin E oil 1/8 teaspoon vanilla extract

Slowly heat beeswax, coconut oil, and vitamin E oil until melted. Stir in the vanilla extract then cool

13.) Vanilla Lip Balm

1 TBL Petroeum Jelly 1 TBL Aloe Vera Gel 1 1/2 tsp coconut oil 1/2 tsp vanilla

Heat in double boiler (or microwave) then pour into container to cool.

14.) Candle Wax Lip Balm

1/2 a teaspoon of melted candle wax.
2 teaspoons of Olive Oil.
1/2 a teaspoon of Shea Butter or you can also add Cocoa Butter. 1/2 a teaspoon of Honey and any flavor of oil to taste.
one vitamin E capsule to preserve the Lip Balm

15.) Eyeshadow Lip Balm

Take an eyeshadow break it up and mix it with vaseline or beeswax. For a glossy shine, use an irridescent or glittery eyeshadow. White/silver/ grey glossys are best.

16.) Cocoa Butter Lip Gloss

1/2 tsp grated Beeswax
1 tsp cocoa butter

1 tsp almond oil, or olive
Melt all together by means of waterbath (put in a cup & set in sink of hot water) and then put into a lip balm container

**this is a butter recipe if you want something glossy but not too.. slick :)

17.) Castor Oil Lip Balm

3 oz castor oil
1.5 cocoa butter
1.5 beeswax
Melt in microwave. Add oil. Stir. Pour into containers.

18.) Sweet Balm/Gloss

2 tsp beeswax
1 tsp honey
7 tsp castor oil or jojoba or sweet almond oil
1/8 tsp. Flavor oil

Melt the oil and beeswax together in a little pan over low heat until the beeswax is melted. Take off the stove and then add in your honey and whisk it all together. When the mixture is nearly cool add in your flavor oil, mix it up again and then pour into your lip balm container. Since this comes out to be more like a gloss you can always add more beeswax to it so that it is a little harder. Maybe another 1/2 tsp would do it.

19.) Heal Sores Balm

3 oz almond oil
2 tsp pure honey
1/2 oz beeswax
1 tsp tea tree oil
Melt all together and stir while cooling.

20.) Quick & Easy Lip Balm

Spoon full of vasiline in a cup (you dont even need to heat it) . Add some honey (depending on how sweet you want it).
Mix together or whip. Lip stick color shavings for color.

To solidify faster after putting it in a container, submerse it in a cup of ice water or put it in the freezer until solid.

21.) Hemp Oil Lip Balm

3 T coconut oil 1 T castor oil
1 T sunflower oil

1 T hemp seed oil
1 T beeswax
1 T honey
Essential Oil to taste (I use peppermint)

Melt the wax, and coconut oil together (I use the microwave)
Add the honey and heat a little. Stir constantly and add your sunflower and caster oil. As the mixture begins to thicken add the hempseed oil and your choice of essential oil. STIR CONTANTLY until it thickens.

22.) Peppermint Lip Balm

2 Tbsp petroleum jelly
1 tspn beeswax
10-14 drops peppermint essential oil

In a small pot, melt the petroleum jelly, then add beeswax.
When melted, remove from heat and add peppermint essential oil. Pour into a lip pot and cool.

23.) Nude Lip Balm Trendy..

1/4 tsp. of aloe vera lotion
1/4 tsp. of your color of foundation 1 tbsp. of vaseline

Mix together in a small bowl with a cotton swab. You can even skip the aloe vera lotion if you want.

24.) Fruity Lip Gloss --Made with Kool-Aid!

2 tbsp. solid shortening
1 tbsp. fruit-flavored powdered drink mix (Kool-Aid) 35 mm plastic film container

Mix shortening and drink mix together in a small microwave-safe container until smooth. Place container in the microwave on high for 30 seconds until mixture becomes a liquid. Pour the mixture into a plastic film container or any other type of small airtight container. Place the fruity lip gloss mixture in the refrigerator for 20 to 30 minutes or until firm.

25.) Cinnamon Lip Gloss

2 tablespoons petroleum jelly
1/4 teaspoon lipstick, any color
4 drops cinnamon oil
Place petroleum jelly in small microwave container. Top with lipstick. Microwave for 20-30 seconds on High power (100%), or until mixture has softened. Blend well. Mix in cinnamon. Store in small container.

26.) Hard Candy Lip Gloss

2 Tbsp petroleum jelly

1 tspn beeswax

2-3 pieces of your favorite hard candy (jolly ranchers work great!)
In a small pot (or micorwave), melt the petroleum jelly, hard candy and beeswax. Pour into a lip container and cool.

In a microwave, melt about eight chocolate chips with about four tablespoons of cocoa butter and 1/4 teaspoon of olive oil. Stir at 20-second intervals until the chocolate melts and the product is well mixed. Place in small containers and refrigerate until hardened. Use as needed. Makes a great gift, too!

27.) Cocoa Butter Minty Lip Balm

1-1/2 parts cocoa butter
1-1/2 parts grated beeswax
3 parts edible vegetable oil of your choice
(almond, apricot kernel, avocado,
extra virgin olive, hemp seed, jojoba, kukui
nut, macadamia nut, castor all work well... but
keep in mind if you plan on selling lip balm or
giving as a gift, that some people are allergic to
nut oils). Spearmint and/or peppermint
flavoring oil Melt the cocoa butter and beeswax
slowly and carefully in a microwave, or over a
double boiler on the stove until melted. Add oil
and stir well. Add spearmint or peppermint
flavoring oils, or both, a few drops at a time, to
taste. Gently reheat if needed. Cool slightly
before pouring into containers. To test
consistency, place
a drop on a spoon and set in the refrigerator to
cool for a few minutes. Test on your lips. For a
softer lip balm, add more oil. For a harder lip
balm, add more beeswax.

28.) Chocolate Lip Gloss

1 1/2 tsp grated cocoa butter
1/2 tsp coconut oil
1/8 tsp vitamin E oil
1/4 tsp grated chocolate or 3 small chocolate
chips
In a double boiler or microwave heat the cocoa
butter, coconut oil, and vitamin E oil until
melted. Stir in the chocolate chips and keep
stirring until melted and well blended Pour into
small container and allow to cool before using

29.) Beeswax Lip Balm

2 tablespoons beeswax
1 tablespoon coconut oil
Melt the ingredients over a double boiler. Pour into a container while still hot since it will harden as it cools. Makes about 1/4 cup.

30.) Cocoa Butter Minty Lip Balm

1-1/2 parts cocoa butter
1-1/2 parts grated beeswax
3 parts edible vegetable oil of your choice (almond, apricot kernel, avocado, extra virgin olive, hemp seed, jojoba, kukui nut, macadamia nut, castor all work well... but keep in mind if you plan on selling lip balm or giving as a gift, that some people are allergic to nut oils)
Spearmint and/or peppermint flavoring oil.

Melt the cocoa butter and beeswax slowly and carefully in a microwave, or over a double boiler on the stove until melted. Add oil and stir well. Add spearmint or peppermint flavoring oils, or both, a few drops at a time, to taste. Gently reheat if needed. Cool slightly before pouring into containers. To test consistency, place a drop on a spoon and set in the refrigerator to cool for a few minutes. Test on your lips. For a softer

lip balm, add more oil. For a harder lip balm, add more beeswax.

All Natural Leg Wax Recipe (Sugaring)

Most of us have seen the infomercials and seen the different leg sugaring products at the drugstore. It's so simple to make yourself and so inexpensive that you'll always make your own!

Sugar Leg Wax

2 C sugar
1/4 C lemon juice
1/4 C water
2 tbsp vegetable glycerine
waxing cloth strips (buy at the drugstore) OR use strips of linen cut to the size of these strips
wooden popsicle sticks (to stir the wax and to apply)

Combine all ingredients in a saucepan. Stir frequently while heating to 250 degrees F or softball stage. Pour into jars and cover with lids. If you use plastic jars, you'll be able to microwave this mixture instead of heating it on the stove. That's it!! You just made your own leg wax/sugar that you'd pay $20 for in the stores!

To use the Sugar Wax:

Heat in the microwave for ten seconds on high. Using a wooden stir stick, stir VERY well. It should be warm but not HOT. Please be very careful when heating up this wax - it's very easy to burn yourself.

If the wax isn't warm enough, place it back in the microwave for five seconds, and stir again. Remember, this is hot sugar syrup- if it gets too hot you'll be badly burned.

Lightly powder the area to be treated. Spread a thin layer of the wax on in the same direction as the hair grows. Apply the waxing cloth strip over the applied wax, and rub down well to get the wax to stick to the cloth. Pull your skin taut, and in one quick motion pull the fabric off of your skin AGAINST the direction of hair growth. Continue with the other areas of your leg or wherever you're waxing.

When you're done waxing a complete area, rub in lotion, aloe vera gel (fresh is best) or oil to soothe your legs.

You can use the homemade waxing strips again if you soak it in soapy water to dissolve the sugar off the fabric and then toss it in with

your wash as normal.

THANK YOU FOR ORDER

BUY VOL. 1
BUY VOL. 2

CPSIA information can be obtained
at www.ICGtesting.com
Printed in the USA
BVHW071346270421
605946BV00002B/629